GOLDEN HILL

Teddy Twoface

ISBN: 1530083389
ISBN 13: 9781530083381

PROLOGUE

By definition a prologue is a section that is supposed to introduce the upcoming work. I am not quite sure how to introduce this one, its kind of complicated. I came straight from a psych ward for 10 days to this rehab where you are going to read all about it. How did I get to that psych ward? Well that's a story for a different time. Just a little back-story, I was fucking out of control. Manic as fuck, I don't even remember checking myself into the hospital. I did it in a drug induced subconscious state. I couldn't sleep and stumbled into my parents room telling them sleep isn't coming and I desperately want it to. They took me to the hospital where they took one look at me and thought I was over dosing. My mother told them to take a look at my medical record so before they could treat me for ODing they realized I was just extremely fucked up and in a manic state. The evil demon called manic-depressive illness or bipolar was unleashed and that fucker had a good grasp on my soul. I'll never know what I said to those doctors but it couldn't have been good because when I woke up from my drug coma I had a nurse staring at me. I was put on 1 on 1 security watch for the next four days. Well I'm not going to delve more into this time in my life because that's for a different book to discuss. This book solely focuses on my time in rehab and the journey that ensued. Fair warning now, if you are sensitive to curse words, there's plenty.

If you're sensitive to the truth, you probably shouldn't read this book. If you think you have a problem with drugs, alcohol or mental illness most definitely read this book. This is my journey with all the above. It's a personal memoir. I am not here to preach and tell you how to live your life that's completely up to you but if my mistakes and newfound wisdom can assist you in making better choices know how happy that makes me. I truly debated publishing this very personal book because it exposes all aspects of my life but in the end I would rather take that risk if it means there is a possibility it can help just one person.

Just to set the time, this book begins with my first day in rehab after being in a mental ward for 10 days. At this point, I know I am taking a semester off from school and my return in the fall is completely intertwined with every single future decision I make from this point on. Eyes are watching my every single move. So smile, its all good or at least it needs to be perceived as so.

So here it is, day one

Well here goes nothing, enjoy fuckers.

LAST DAY IN MENTAL WARD JOURNAL ENTRY

And it ends here, or at least this chapter in my life's book. I'll be departing from my mental ward family and entering a land of unknown called Golden Hill. Hmmm how does this make me feel? Happy, sad, excited, nervous, conflicted but most importantly prepared. I'm ready for this next step. I want to further my progression. That is classic me mentality. Always striving for the number one spot, even if it's for the most mentally improved award. I'm going to embrace my reality and straight murder whatever Golden Hill has to offer. If its yoga, I'll be the best stretcher. If it's AA, I'll be the kid taking notes and raising his hand. Too much progress has been made to relapse. Remember that as you move forward dude and don't ever forget that truth. As I depart from this place, I am showered with wishes of good fortune and luck. Now lets get it straight, it's not that I am refusing their prayers but rather deflecting them. Success during this step in my journey came from me not God so I don't need his blessing. Don't get me wrong, its nice to have, I just don't need it, I got all I need inside of me. Success does not rely on luck but rather will power. I have the will, the pure determination, beast mode Marshawn Lynch style, to complete this chapter with sangfroid. It's who I am and It's how I have always done things. If I'm going in there, I'm coming in with swagger and confidence. Hide yo kids and more importantly your daughters because Teddy Twoface is coming to Golden Hill.

DENIAL: WEEK ONE

Day 1 I'm not quite sure how to start this one because I'm truly at a loss of words. Coming from my caged psych ward to Golden Hill, the juxtaposition may cause head trauma. The living arrangements closely resemble hotels, the food is supposedly fantastic and all the staff is incredibly nice. You know that type of nice where it's almost eerie? Yah, that's what this place is. They told me I'm the first kid to ever come into this place with such a big smile on my face. They probably thought I was truly insane. It's just baffling to me that a place like this exists on this Earth. After the nurse was done asking her list of mundane psychiatric questions, I'm left alone in my hotel suite to write and read to my pleasure. Perceive me as insane, but I think I'm going to enjoy my forced stay here at Golden Hill. Or am I? Who fucking knows? Not me, that's for sure.

I am now a firm believer in the saying, "You have to have some rainy days in order in enjoy the sunny ones". The minutest things to me today felt orgasmic since my standards of living were so low in the hospital aka, the mental asylum. For example, the shower was steamy hot and the pressure was almost too hard. No more flooding, limp dick pressure showers for me. It's just more physical exemplifications of my ever- growing progress towards mental sanity. I didn't even flitch or mind when they came knocking at 5 in the morning to take my blood. Damn, I must really be insane.

DAY 2

Day two and I have completed my daily goal setting by 11 o'clock. Let me explain how it works at Golden Hill. First, you first get placed in the "Lodge", a detox unit where everyone goes first to be examined and prepped for their future houses. There are so many different type of houses it reminds me of Hogwarts. I hope I'm in Gryffindor! The people and stories I've heard in the first 24 hours of being in the detox unit were incredible. I'll never forget the people and words they imparted on me. Detox patients are different than your usual psych patients. Detox patients, for the most part, are all there mentally, they just have addictions. What we all have in common though is we all are sick with a disease most of us don't want to admit we have. The lodge, as beautiful as it is, has the lingering smell of cigarette smoke. Patients were allowed breaks to smoke sometimes and that made them exuberant. I loved these guys. They were raw, real manly men. Cursed like manic people and had humor that spoke of their long journeys, usually dry and crude. It was all so honest, so real, so accepting. It was almost a shame I was being transferred to a new house. They call it Scativa house or as I like to call it, "the Sativa house". It's the little things like that, that get me by. I should have known, living in a house of alcoholics and addicts that this name would stick.

One person I met in the lodge, named Hank, really made an impression on me. He had a raspy voice, white and brown scraggly beard and unkempt clothes. I deduced from his lack of participation in smoke breaks that his raspy voice probably had to do with the large noticeable scar around his neck. Twenty minutes into a one on one talk with him I learned so much about him, about myself, and about the time period he grew up in. He proceeded to tell me that he tried to take his own life, hence the raspy voice. He radiated joy however, as this man wanted to live. After he failed to end his life he decided that to end a life is the most cowardly thing to do. He said, "Life is too damn hard, death should be easy". I'll never forget that line and I'll sure as fuck never forget Hank.

And now my journey continues to the Sativa house. I was given a binder full of organized tabs and four books ranging from Alcoholics Anonymous to Living Sober. Ok Golden Hill, I see you. You are clearly not fucking around. See, Golden Hill is a dual diagnosis program. it's a hospital as well as a rehabilitation center. I'm not an alcoholic or addicted to drugs, I like weed you caught me! I'm feeling like a lot of this is going to be OD but I'll take it with a grain of salt. With a promotion into my new frat house, I have regained much independence. I get to roam an open campus and use amenities like the gym. Time to get swoll. It seriously feels like my first day of sleep away camp except this isn't Timberlake, this is camp for recovering degenerates where the deranged can congregate and get better together.

I had this thought today, every tool for me to succeed for the next 28 days is smack in front of my face. Straight up, I'm going to use them to reach an enlightenment of sorts, become content with who I am and where I am. I'm going to be living a perfect 28 sober days and following my progression, I'm going to reach levels my body has never reached before, physically and mentally. I'm excited. It's like my secret mission. I'm like 007; mission is to reach nirvana in 28 days straight bond style with swagger and poise. Except I'm pretty sure if I fuck anyone I get kicked out, so every facet of Bond minus his game with ladies, for now at least.

I just finished my first NA meeting and my head is spinning, my heart is hurting and I'm fighting back tears. That my friends should set the tone of where this is going. A lot of things were said and a lot of things resounded with me. I am not going to be the guy that goes to one meeting and proclaims he's seen God's penis. I'm here to tell the truth and nothing but. First off, "One is too many and 1000 is never enough". Fuck me. That one quote really got to me. Do I love weed? Yes. Is one bong rip enough? Never. Am I addicted to weed? Am I an addict? As you can see these thoughts are real and prevalent. More importantly is this notion of in and out. All the speakers said it tonight. "I've been in and out of rehabs 30 times". That thought scares the shit out of me. I can't fathom another stay in a mental ward. I know I have bipolar and it is the definition of cycles but I refuse to let it reoccur over and over again. Nah, fuck you, I won't. I am going to end this inevitable detrimental cycle. I am going to break the wheel Khalessi style. Addicts have three inevitable outcomes: jail, institutions and death but somewhere in that fucking handbook says something about will power and that ladies and gents is something I have. Call it a disease if you want to use terms being tossed around nowadays but I'm breaking the cycles and you can go fuck yourself if you doubt me.

DAY 3

1 3 days sober, three days into the new program. Aight ladies and gents we have ourselves a ball game. So far my secret mission to become a Zhenren as the Doaists like to describe an enlightened individual is going swimmingly. Matter of fact, I'm about to swim and hit the weights for the first time since I've been here. I have so much testosterone built up its going to feel therapeutic to release it all naturally.

Yep, I was completely correct. Nothing better than a needed pump. That sounds douchey but I mean it in a therapeutic way. The gym center includes a pool, changing room and a mini bodega. A bodega. Yep, I know it's ludicrous. To quote Annie, yes the musical, "I think I'm going to like it here". After my first full scheduled day of Scativa activities I'm left physically and emotionally exhausted. I had my first AA meeting and boy do I have some fundamental disagreements. Well, that likely stems from me not being an alcoholic. That's not me, never was, and if had to choose for life it would be weed every time. Now here comes the intellectual sparring. The speaker droned on about his personal journey and how he overcame his illness. Before we begin, it should be noted that I highly respect this man and all he has done for himself and others. However, he preached finding a higher power and it was only then we could find salvation. Now hold the fuck up. What? Let's pull the full quote from the big book, "Lack of power that was our dilemma. We had to find a power which we could live, and it had to be a power greater than ourselves. Obviously. But where and how were we to find this Power" (45). So, ok. Like in the quote it says, "Obviously". We are meant to conclude that the power we need comes from a religious god. This is the root of the disagreement, for many reasons. First and foremost, I do not believe in God. AH! Yes, I said it and if I happen to be wrong oh do I have some choice words for the big guy upstairs. I believe in fate. Side note, do you know who ended up becoming my roommate? HANK! The first guy I met in detox. Although we are around 30 years apart we have so much in common it hurts. Is this fate showing me a possible mirror older version of myself? Maybe, I'm not quite sure. So yes back to AA, they preach giving over power to a higher power due to the obvious lack of self-power. This is where I object most strongly. Everything that has and will happen will come through me and only me, not God. I have the ultimate power to pick up a bottle of tequila or not. The thought of giving my power over to someone else, even if it's this God fellow, scares the shit out of me because ultimately I'm conquering this, not him. I haven't seen him come down from his perch and intervene positively. If anything that fucker has been sitting idle during my follies and probably getting a chuckle or two. I am a man who seeks the truth. I am a realist and a spiritual man no doubt, but don't tell me to give up my power to anyone. How fucking dare you! I'll do as I please motha fucka and in the end the result might be the same or it might not. All I know is all power and choice is going to come through me and only me.

Go figure, after my rant we have back –to-back AA meetings and this one was heavily god orientated. Now just being who I am,

I'm always asking questions. Did some higher power do this to try to drive a specific point into my brain in order to switch my perspective? At the end of the day, I affirmed some major concepts of my moral code. A) I don't believe in God. B) People who do can be tolerated and some simply cannot. C) There is no higher power higher than you.

Now I can rest easy. Goodnight ladies and gents, believe whatever you please, as is your innate right but it's also mine to write about how dumb you all truly sound giving away your courage to a nameless, faceless higher power.

DAY 4

My day started at 7:30 AM in a very unique and interesting way. If you ever want to wake up naturally try engaging in an intellectual conversation. That's what Hank did with me this morning. I could tell so many issues weighted him down. All it took was, "How ya feeling Hank?" to open up the floodgates. He is the nicest man who has had all the wrong things happen to him: nasty divorce, lawsuits, cheating girlfriend and failed suicide. We discussed his issues and he conveyed all his problems with the judicial system, religion and the ills of choosing the wrong woman. After it all, I sat in my bed pondering where this man's honest fault was and I couldn't find one. I gave him my advice, "You need to let karma run its course and not let these thoughts ruin you". After I said this, his face dropped and I'll never forget what he said next. In his raspy voice, "In all my years and experience I've never met someone with so much clarity". Clarity you say, well Hank, its easy to see clearly once you awake from a mental halt and drug binge hibernation.

Well ladies and gents once again, age is just a number. I just finished my first yoga session and as expected, I loved it. My Siddhartha side was finally able to be released. It felt refreshing. I got to naturally release all these tension points and after I felt new and clean, similarly to waking up after a nap. I can see why people love this shit, straight addicted to it. As I stretched my way through my first class, the teacher continued to emphasize our minds and what/why we were thinking thoughts, if any at all. I loved it. I stayed in the moment as much as I could. Only issue I can foresee is that the stretching, flexible girls in front of me are going to quickly take me out of my present moment. Well I guess in a sense that is my present moment. Ah but the yoga gods have me by the balls, they found out my weakness. Flexible girls are going to do me in one day if I slip up. That, and weed. If I could only conquer women and weed I could actually become a Buddhist monk.

I just had another AA meeting. Going into it with the same attitude, expecting to gain more fuel for my intellectual sparring but, I was wrong. It started to happen after my boy Zach raised his hand. He proclaimed that as you go deeper and deeper into this process the more you reveal about yourself. Fuck man, he was right. There were levels to this shit to use Meek Mills lingo. Spiritual levels, emotional levels, realistic levels and then my hand rose. My mind was shocked as no command was given to move my arm. I stated for the first time, "Hi, my name is Teddy and I am an addict". When you share it aloud it has a profound effect. It confirms the thoughts that race in your head. I shared that I didn't per say have an issue with alcohol but I did with weed however, and if you substituted them the whole AA book made a hell of a lot more sense. After I shared I was applauded and after the meeting I was hugged. That got me higher than any bong rip or spliff.

Flying high, I went to my next meeting which happened to be an AA meeting run by a girl named Anastasia. Banging name. I already got good vibes from her. As she told her story, I found myself more intrigued and less tired. This is what I am discovering is the essence of AA for me personally. All about relating to stories and applying them to my plight. Her words captivated me, using phrases like, "chasing euphoria" and "bubble of insanity". I could really relate and then she said she went to Wisconsin. I immediately raised my Wisco beanie and said, "Fellow badger". She laughed and very matter of fact responded, "And here we are". Damn, don't even know how to feel after that one. Well-played Anastasia. Her journey to sobriety was no easy feat but here she was now, sober. Her closing statement was she switched professions because she wanted to fixate on helping others. She wasn't grandiose. All she wanted was to effect one person and then another and so on. That's where I could really relate. This book isn't a guidebook for the deranged to find sanity. It's just a book, one that speaks to the truths of my long journey to mental stability. You want a good read? Keep reading. If not, I don't really give a fuck.

DAY 5

15 days sober. That has a nice ring to it. Down to keep the forward progression. Today, the first person that showed me around the Scativa house departed on his journey to sobriety. I wish you the best of luck my man. As we exchanged info, I came to the realization that this dude is currently my only sober friend. I aim to fix that. He's a celebrity cook doing quite well for himself and he's sober as an ox. He creates this aura of positive vibes, vibes that I would like to surround myself in.

And surrounding me with positive energy is exactly what I did today. It started in a surprisingly non-positive way. I'm not sure why, but I partook in having a cigarette. Actually, I do know why I did it. It was right after breakfast and Jake, my boy, had a menthol Newport. Fuck it, what's living a balanced lifestyle if you don't have one sin to balance. From then on, it was all positive. We had meditation where we read a beautiful passage about birds chirping in the morning. Everyone had his or her own interpretation. While some viewed it negatively, I viewed it positively. It talked about "Predawn darkness" and its inevitability to turn to light. It reminded me of my manic days of staying up all night drugged out. Hearing those birds chirp was your pat on the back for accomplishing your nightly binge and that it was time to start your next day of delirium.

I went directly to the gym after to play basketball, lift, swim and eventually try Tai Chi for the first time. I smoked some fools 2 v 2 but I had to keep in mind my competition. This wasn't the NBA this was a mental hospital. I then lifted and hopped into the pool. The poolroom, surrounded by all glass, is incredibly serene. All alone, I slid into the warmth. Doing laps centered me, it was calming and I was instantly addicted, classic addict behavior. It is a different type of aerobic activity that I haven't engaged in quite some time. I found a lot of swimming strokes reassembled what I later learned in Tai Chi. All very natural and flowing. Swimming, with the body's air deficiency, forces you to stay in the moment. The correlations to the Chi and more broadly Daoism is actually quite strong. The Tai Chi itself was superb. I could tangibly feel the energy flow and dissipate from my body. Yes, the force is strong with this one. Again, I was instantly hooked. When I created my "Chi ball" I could feel the sensation between my hands, it was real. If this was real, I wonder what else those wise Asian fuckers are keeping from us. Not keeping from us, we are just too ignorant in the West to have an open mind towards it. Not me, I'm game. At 19, I'm going to be just fine. The progress and Chi said that- not me -ladies and gents.

The latter portion of my day was highly AA driven. Our house group fixated again on the principle of being in AA and not believing in God. I finally got some answers I was content with, one coming from Hank. He shared that with his near death experience he did not see any white light. No pearly gates, just the flashing of one's life. He explained his ideology that there is no god but there is something tying us all together called fate, destiny and coincidence. Yes, Hank, preach on you atheist you. My second answer actually came much later after the meeting. I engaged in a philosophical talk with a staff member who works at the gym. We share common interests in Buddhism and Daoism. I explained to him my dilemma. His analogy that followed was brilliant. I told him god couldn't be my higher power since I didn't believe in his existence. He told me to turn to nature, specifically the sun. He said look up. You can see it and feel its warmth. It connects us all; it gives plants energy, animal's food and humans the ability to sustain life. Aight stoner looking gym dude, I feel you hard. This made me smile. I was content.

DAY 6

So I can finally put in words what my mission here really is, besides staying sober of course, it's to pursue happiness. True, unadulterated, pure natural happiness. I want it more than the dankest nug and the nicest Illadelph. It's because of my acknowledgment of this that I have the utmost faith I'll complete my goal.

My day, unlike any other thus far, was not filled with sunshine and rainbows. Lemme tell you the series of events. It started wonderfully spiritual because I partook in the "early bird" AA meeting that starts at 7 at a chapel a short drive away. Watching the sunrise, I see on display my higher power. The AA meeting really isn't worth delving into; it had some great analogies and I found a temporary sponsor. When I got back I did my becoming standard procedure: Bike, lift, swim. I Love how at peace I feel afterwards. Then things took a nosedive out of left field. During a small class the notion of belonging here was brought up with my social worker. She questioned if I still truly needed to be here, mind you this is only day 6, less than a week. That really fucked with my mentality and eventually was the catalyst of an argument with my mother when she came to visit. My clarity was temporarily fogged but like any mirror sometimes you just need to buff it out when it fogs, funny because in the end you are left with a clearer mirror, similarly to my mind.

With my spirits hampered I went to my last meeting of the day, NA. Once again, they have yet to fail me. To start, one of the speakers was wearing a Sons of Anarchy t-shirt, red wood original homie, good looks. The speaker and his proceeding story will forever be positively burned into my memory banks. He spoke with raw emotion and power. I could feel him staring into my soul and I bet everyone felt like that. He told us his war story of addiction to all drugs and he did not discriminate. "If I wasn't vomiting, it wasn't strong enough". He told us it got to the point where he hated it. Hated to do the drugs and knew it was bad but couldn't prevent it. That was disease taking over. Man, I know it's not crack but that's how I feel with weed. This man watched his brother die, been to jail four times and still he stood. He preached a day at a time, just for today, be sober and your life will slowly start to change. He is now a father to a five-year-old living in a house he built with his own hands. He also works with a school with children with special needs. You know who are and if you ever end up reading this know you A) changed my shitty mood and B) changed my life for the better.

DAY 7

Been officially one week and I have made some serious short term and broader revelations. To begin where I left off yesterday, I confirmed some major concepts. One is that I am hundo P seeing this through till the end. I belong in this 28- day program and I am no quitter so fuck it, I'll embrace the pampered, luxurious rehab for what it is. Secondly, I had a thought that my purpose here isn't solely focused on me. Take the plane analogy, you first need to place the air mask on yourself when the plane is crashing and then you can assist others. That's where I am now. Lemme tell you how I arrived at this mentality switch.

It starts with Grace's story but truly goes much deeper. At lunch this sweet young girl named Grace sat next to me. She told me she got in a little trouble last night, and I asked how? She was feeling stressed so to cope, she dunked her head in the river. She laughed as she told it and told me everyone perceived her as insane. I laughed right back and said, "No, you're not crazy you're just unique". We all have our own methods of coping, who the fuck are they to judge? She left lunch happy and told me, "Wow, you are seriously a great dude". She was jealous of how Zen I seemed, so I told her I have plenty and could give her some whenever she needed. I later told my mom about this exchange over the phone and I could hear her getting choked up. She reminded me of my childhood nickname, "Human Prozac" and my skill of lightening any dark situation. She told me that skill never left me and that it was in every bone of my body. I hung up that phone call feeling very confident in my abilities.

So back to my legitimate regimented routine. I again went to the early bird AA meeting and this time I donated a dollar. They provide coffee and donuts so I didn't see a problem in a donation as long as it wasn't going directly to "god". Plus, I took a monster shit in the churches nice ass bathroom. I see where the money REALLY goes. I didn't mind, I was actually quite the opposite. I was appreciative "god" gave me this nice bathroom to decimate. Whatta blessing. The actual content of the meeting was interesting and relevant. It was about the AA slogans. It was comforting to hear from my peers that they also had an issue with the whole "god" thing. The slogans that didn't involve "god" I could identify with. It talked about how we are not responsible for our first thought, even if it jeopardized our sobriety. It talked a lot about living in the now and remembering that when life gets "life-y" one must breathe and learn to cope. My main revelation from the meeting was to use the slogans as reminders for greater concepts, to put aside expectations since they tend to bring upon letdowns. To quote my homie Siddhartha, "Expectations are resentments in waiting". Ahh, I'm in a good place mentally as you can see.

My courses today were very enlightening. I learned new ways to cope with anxiety. They call them DBT skills. I embrace any new skill or any new knowledge as a matter of fact. I got to meet with my doc and discuss my meds and we, or really I, created a long term plan to wean me off the negative drugs (Ambien, Seroquel) and remain on the positive ones (Depakote and Risperdal). I am so on top of my shit even the doctor was impressed. It's my body, my temple, so it makes sense.

I ended my day with a positive AA meeting where the speaker told her fascinating story of destruction and recovery. After I had a cig with the boys and when I say my boys I truly mean brothers. We all have become incredibly close. Guess that's just the product of sticking 16 drug addicts all going through the same shit all living under the same roof. Goodnight Sativa house, stay beautiful.

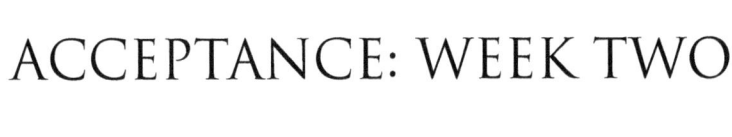

ACCEPTANCE: WEEK TWO

DAY 8

"Nearly every serious emotional problem can be seen as a case of misdirected instinct". Hell of a quote to be dropped on you at 7:30 AM in the early bird AA meeting. I digged it hard. It's hitting on the concept that emotions, especially rash ones, more often than not, lead to an eventual path of self-destruction. My past is over flowing with emotion. No wonder I self-imploded.

Now that my ears and mind are open wider than double doors, I'm learning so many integral skills that I can apply to my fight with sobriety. After the whirly bird, I had a day heavily focused on spirituality. That's how Wednesdays work here at the Hill. It started in a group called "Creative Spirituality" aka creative open mic for anyone who wanted to participate. Since it was my first time attending, I decided to be an active pacifist and take notes, and notes I took. My boys Maximus and Arthur Duke (stage names) wrote and performed a song called, "My Friends". It hit me right in the feels. It was sung by Arthur Duke, deep and soulful voice, and played perfectly by Maximus. It tells a tale of misery, using nature motifs to explain his isolation. His friends would, "call his name" but he always ends up missing the ride. Really powerful shit, but what really got me came from left field and it didn't even demonstrate depth or creativity. This sweet, young girl got up on the podium and said she was going to read, "Twas' a Night before Christmas". Fuck, here comes the waterworks. It evoked such strong feelings for me because every Christmas eve my parents used to read the story to my brother and I. I cried like a little girl, the nostalgic ties were too overwhelming. So many more brave souls shared their poems and songs, quotes original and not, were being dropped left and right. A 14 year old sang an original song dealing with the effects of burning bridges and the irreversibility of said actions. Once burned and charred, they can never be quite the same. Concepts much too complex for girls of their age were being demonstrated in front of my eyes and I was shocked, dumbfounded, impressed beyond belief and left with a dropped jaw.

I then segued into a meditation group. I've only really tried it a handful of times but this time I really fucking nailed it. I focused on my breathing and refused to slip into sleep and more importantly slip into another moment other than the present. After the 45 minutes, I slowly opened my eyes, wow I was more awake than ever and felt more rested than an awakening coma patient. I was able to access a part of my brain I didn't know existed. I have spiritually activated the full capacity of my brain and now that I felt what it feels like I'm never going to give that up. Meditation naturally increases serotonin levels, similarly to what drugs do to the brain. Meditation over molly ladies and gents.

DAY 9

S o it's Christmas Eve and I'm here. The honest truth is A) I couldn't be more content being here with the people I'm with and B) I truly forgot it was even Christmas Eve. My only reminder was at night when the boys put on "The Christmas Story". Whatta classic.

I spent most of the day in reflection. That's probably why I forgot about all the Christmas hype. I made lists in my journal ranging from reminders for when I get released, to stay away from trigger points, to lists of girls I've been with. There will always be one girl who will remain at the top of the list regardless of whatever happens in life, that's just my heart, its still infected with childhood love. Well anyway, boredom is the devil's playground and murders sobriety so I tend to occupy my brain with the present or contemplating the past. I also made lists of future stocks I want to invest in and day dreamed about opening up my own clothing store.

My course part of the day was very mentally and spiritually appealing. We watched part of an HBO special "Addiction" and it was quite powerful. It hit on points about public perception and the misunderstanding that alcoholism isn't a disease. Oh, it most certainly is and a fucking powerful one. I gathered that public perception leads to misunderstanding of the broader issues at hand. The ignorance of the masses pollutes and affects everyone, in the complete negative side of the spectrum.

Then I was informally introduced to Kristin Johnson, a writer and addict who wrote a book called "Guts" and guts is something this lady had myriad amounts of. She instantly became a role model for me, someone to strive to be like. She said powerful quotes about relating addiction to the black plague. She was pressured to be silent but she did the complete opposite. Go Kristin, silence your haters. Tell your story and tell it however the fuck you please. You showed me I'm not alone in this fight, we are all in this together, supporting each other. We are all in the same lifeboat and this is not the Titanic, we will not sink. Life will get hard and temptations will naturally lie ahead and have a place along the journey of life, but I don't care. It's my world now fuckers and I aim to set it straight. There are triggers in this world, no doubt, but I will not take the cowardly path and squeeze my index finger on the metaphoric gun pointed to my temple.

DAY 10

"There's nothing in this world I wouldn't do to be a better father to you, so lemme show you" my dad said through his soft choked up voice. Today started feeling a lot like Christmas or as much as it could when you're in rehab. The early bird meeting was charged with spirituality and jolly moods. The nature I was immersed in was tangibly serene. I was in a jolly mood as well so I donated 2 dollars, Merry Christmas. We later segued into meditation where it was guided by mountain motifs. I focused hard on staying present and the outcome was surly bliss and serenity. Little did I know that would be my last taste of such feelings.

When my family arrived I could tell something was wrong. My dad tends to wear his emotions on his sleeve. I pulled him aside and began to pry. He told me he was done. At 51, he was done drinking and that he was going to join me in sobriety. He warned and reminded me of our previous talk yesterday when I coined the term "sober-ish". He explained that was not the way he was going to go about it. I respected his honesty. He was crying the whole time he was talking to me. I stayed strong for him and thanked him for joining me in the good fight. It was emotional but we were just scrapping the barrel of emotional magnitude I just didn't know it yet, the worst was yet to come.

The facade of happiness and normalcy overtook my family as we chucked the pigskin and laughed but that eventually faded. It was time to face the elephant in the room. I had so many pent up emotions that I needed to address with them so that's what I did. I didn't care that it was Christmas or fearful of how emotional this talk would get, all I knew was that it had to happen. I explained my greater understanding of my bipolar illness and gave a general sense of how to protect myself. This purpose of this conversation was meant to be me explaining my perspective and the time would later come for them to respond. That didn't stop my mom from butting in on everything I had to say but whatever. I explained to them the triggers that drove me to the point of insanity and how they all played a crucial role in it. All three of them, my mother, father and brother, sat in silent guilt for a while. I pointed out the effects that my family including my brother has inflicted upon me. I then went on my final heart wrenching rant. I emphatically spoke about my disease and how it could be potentially stronger than I. That if I were mistreated I would surely die by my own devices or external variables. I reminded them of the terrible side effects of high doses of lithium and xeprexa, medications of my first episode. I made a lifesaving decision to go against the doctors and my family's advice, go to Wisconsin for summer classes and flush all the toxins down the toilet. If it weren't for my bravery I would have done the opposite and crawled atop my roof and jumped. This is about the time in the conversation my mother was streaming tears and begging me to stop. I asked them if they would enjoy a family of 3. They were heart broken. My parents left but before they did we all hugged it out and that's when my father whispered that line into my ear that I will never forget.

I was sad, jumbled up and confused and now depressed. I didn't know how to change my mood but I did know I wanted it to change desperately. I took a walk to the butt hut and smoked a couple cigarettes and listened to old Tupac. That seemed to help a little. On my way back, I past the now gushing river due to previous nights of rainfall, it was beautiful. I stopped to listen and sat by the river. I meditated Siddhartha style and when I was done I felt much more relaxed. When I got back to the house, the boys immediately lifted my spirits. They told me to bring my I-pod and cigs to the butt hut because we were going to have a little party, listening to music, talking and smoking. I was game. For 45 minutes, we all laughed, guys and girls, and chilled until security came and shut us down. Fuck the police, we're straight outta Golden Hill.

DAY 11

Days sober: 21, blackjack! Oh fuck wait, that's a trigger, gambling is bad! Today my day was filled with positivity, no post-Christmas blues for me. I used my Teflon Mind (DBT skill) to observe my thoughts as they passed through and made damn sure the negative ones didn't latch on to my frontal lobe. In one of my more productive classes today, no sarcasm, we watched an episode of Modern Family in order to identify the triggers the characters faced. It was a productive exercise. The exercise was a trigger in itself because up until this moment, I've never watched an episode without my girlfriend, now ex, laying on my chest. This ex played a large role in my life while I was stable and unfortunately when I was manic and I'm proud to say her name didn't even cross my mind as I watched and I found myself laughing my ass off at the scenes I used to watch with her. Later in the day I passed Grace, we had our becoming usual exchange: "We're going to fucking kill it, let's do this". She's just great and I love that girl.

My sponsor, who I've failed to heed his request to call him every day, ran the nightly AA meeting and he promptly called me out on my bullshit. That's the type of shit that doesn't bother me and does the contrary; it reminds me of why I chose him as a sponsor. He shared his story briefly but what hit me was the latter of his share. He cared so much about his family and specifically his daughters that he told us he kisses them as often as he could. That to me makes a man, someone strong enough to speak the truth and show vulnerability. It was all this that accumulated in my big personal share. I shared how I was feeling and how I conquered my depressed episode using DBT skills. I shared with the room that I had such a tough Christmas since I had to clean out my closet and share to my family they were triggers to my mania. I didn't hold back, I told them about how bad it got and how it turned potentially suicidal. After sharing, the room was in a roar filled with clapping and the very pretty girl next to me whispered to me, "Thank you for sharing". Well that alone justified it but it truly felt great to again let it all out. After the meeting was over one of my girlfriends pulled me aside and told me she identified with my story. She also is doing much better and to know my story helped her is going to make me sleep easy tonight.

DAY 12

Today was a day where I'm left in awe, struck by the power of this place and its magical healing powers for anyone who enters through its gates. We watched the Chris Herren documentary and I was taken aback by how powerful it was. This was the first of many similar moments I was going to encounter on this enlightening day. Chris's story was breathtakingly emotional. The man had so much talent; so much he could play NBA games fucked up on opioids and still kill it. I did not think that was cool but quite the opposite. He was living a double life and he knew it. When he finally surrendered and went to rehab after putting his wife and three kids through hell, he was at the start of his journey to recovery. What really struck me was how he was treated in rehab, treated like any other junkie. He described his experience in what they called the "pot sink", a kitchen where he spent 20 days solely washing everyone's dishes. He told the cameras this was where he was forced to face his demons, his disease. What also struck me was his relationship with his oldest son. As he gradually sobered up over the years, he would give his sober AA chips to him. He said that feeling was greater than any trophy he ever received. It quickly reminded me of my own father and his recent decision to live in sobriety. He's only on day three but promised me later on the phone he would continue the tradition Chris Herren started.

My second powerful moment and also moment of gratitude happened when we had an in-house speaker come. He told his captivating story of destruction and redemption but that's not what moved me. What moved me is after when I shared he told me he was bipolar too. He was on lithium for 10 years until it started messing with his kidneys, then started being on Depakote like me. He told me gained 25 lbs from it so that's encouraging! I'll turn it into pure muscle so it's chill. He's living proof though of a success story of someone that has had to battle this potential life threatening mental illness. It gives me immense hope. Bless this man; he's a minister so that's ok to say. Can't say, "God bless" because I can't make demands to the big guy if I've been repetitively shunning the dude. Whatever gets the job done though as long as the end result is the same: happiness, sobriety and success. What really scared the fuck out of me though was after he shared I asked him how he stayed stable all these years, expecting his answer to be medication but I was quite wrong. He said this disease has you by the balls and could grab them at any time. I conveyed how scared that made me but he said he couldn't lie, that I had to honor.

To end my day of emotion, a speaker shared his story at our nightly AA meeting. He had a tough childhood being Japanese and having high expectations for himself along with intense pressure from his family. He felt resentment constantly and due to this he had his first beer at age 12. While his disease was initially under the radar, he has endured a divorce and arrest for three DUI's. He relapsed and started smoking weed every day. He said it helped because it took him out the present moment, I found that interesting. As he told of his recovery he mentioned making amends to his alcoholic father and bipolar mother. The last line he said is what solidified his power of speaking. Through tears and I quote, "I underestimated this program and how it works". Wow, such raw emotion and vulnerability. This is a man I look up to and hope to become half as successful as him. Success defined by not money or materialistic goods but happiness. This man has happiness and that ladies and gents is what I strive for.

DAY 13

My day started with bullshit and the theme stayed constant throughout. It started with the early bird literature. The 24-hour reflection passage used the word "god" 7 times in a short paragraph and the responses from the crowd contained a myriad amount of godly god synonyms. "God is in all of us". Yo, old dude in the back, please speak for your fucking self. They said that god doesn't judge, that's good because my words and actions definitely qualify to be judged. What really set me off is when they said you could bring out god through meditation. No, please don't correlate my higher power of nature and meditation with your white-collar cult. Ok, that was a little harsh it's been a rough day but the meaning behind my words are valid. I did however get some nuggets of wisdom through the meeting. The quote, "perfection is direction and progress is the goal" resonated with me. It was all just eh. So I decided, since I was so opinionated on the subject matter, to share. If you asked my middle school self to voluntarily share his thoughts about religion vs. spirituality in a room filled with 90 people I would have said go fuck yourself. I guess I have outgrown my childhood days of nervousness. Guess I'm just at peace with myself. The coolest part was I proudly admitted that at 19 years old I didn't believe in god, I said it out loud, and people laughed genuinely and after I was fist bumped.

After that share, things continued to drag. I had an anger management class where ironically the teacher was 15 minutes late and I had a below average meeting with my doctor. Then my parents came and completely fucked my day over. The topic of money was brought up, things were said and before long I was frantically scrambling to self-meditate and use all the DBT skills known to mankind. To make matters worse, smoking cigarettes was brought up because that is where they think I'm allocating my funds. My mom always brings up in tears that her father and my grandpa died of lung cancer. That's the shit I can't and won't handle when I'm in rehab for gods (natures) sake. It's all too much. At dinner I stoically told my family that it's becoming evident that they are constant triggers on the negative side of the spectrum. At 19, knowing the fact that the loving supportive family that has nurtured me from the moment my eyes opened for the first time has become constant reminders of the darkest times of my existence is a tough pill to swallow. Tougher than the horse size pills of Depakote I take nightly.

To end my joyous day I get a phone call from a girl who goes to Wisconsin with me. It started off benign and even humorous at times but the inevitable was brought up about our pending status. I guess I expected things to pick up where we left off but I was hypo-manic so I guess that left her with some PTSD. She has some of her own personal issues so it's quite difficult. Women are harder to crack than padlocks my friends. I failed to remember my wise Buddha friend that, "expectations are resentments in waiting". I also failed to stay strong, with my Teflon mind, because after that phone call and the accumulating shit storm, I couldn't shake my emotions. I was not a Teflon don as 50 cent likes to call it, but fuck it, tomorrow will be a better day, it just has to, and it's how karma works, right?

DAY 14

Alcohol this marijuana that, DBT this CBT that, suicide this jails that, sanity this madness that. It was all becoming a recurrent blur. The line between therapeutic and annoying repetitiveness was as well becoming blurred. I guess I just have the halfway done blues. 14 days deep though and I've learned exponentially more in this time span than my two years combined at Wisconsin, yet in some areas I wasn't making any progress.

I still have issues dealing with my family, no AA meeting or speaker is going to be able to change that I know but my hope is I gain the wisdom to be able to not only tolerate but to prosper with their support. I was still irritable with them from yesterday and when my Doc mentioned in passing that he got a frantic message from my mother explaining her fears and the possibility of me slipping into mania again, I almost lost it. Mania?!?! I'm in a fucking rehab on medication I don't even think that's physically possible. It was the way I handled it which made me happy. I called her and explained why this reinforces my lack of trust in this family. I feel constantly scrutinized and judged. What mental state is Teddy in today? Is he a 6? A 7? Or full blown manic? Apparently it was a misunderstanding but my day started with bullshit so I was already cocked to explode. At 6:30 AM, I was told I needed my Risperdal shot so I had to miss the Early Bird AA and when I show up they A) don't have the shot and B) I'm in the wrong place. Bad start to today but I remained that endearing crazy calm that I'm becoming known for. Last aspect of my frustrating day came from the Hill's lazy, not on top of their shit routine. They rarely tell you the full truth and are even more rarely on time for groups. I wouldn't care but they're so anal about us being on time so it's a wicked double standard. Whatever, I'll be like a phoenix and be born again through ashes of frustration, irritability and madness.

Besides all the negatives, I was able to find levity in the Scativa house and the nightly AA meeting. Actually my day started off with intelligible comments from the boys regarding a Ralph Waldo Emerson quote and the importance of picking yourself up when you've fallen. It was one of my boys who started it off. He brought up the idea of karma that he believes he has suffered enough and joy was eventually coming his way. He described cyclical behavior where joy turns to pain, love to hate and poetic words turning acidic. It was eloquently said for someone just speaking their mind. Later in the day he confided in me and told me that I reminded himself of a younger him. I took that to heart because he's someone I strive to be like: wise, soft spoken, a leader and damn handsome.

At the end of the day, it's the individual that determines the value of the 24 hours. I don't need others to change their behavior to ease my feelings. I'm quite content with who I am and where my mental stability lies. Just for today, I'm sane. That is a notion I'll be asking myself and reaffirming for the rest of my life and I'm cool with that.

RECOVERY: WEEK THREE

DAY 15

I lost my notebook today so I'm recalling these events straight off the dome. See the wonders of not smoking weed? The early bird meeting in my mind is I, looking at the second hand tick ever so slowly. I sat next to my newfound friend/fellow addict, Chris. A day prior he pulled me aside and told me he wanted to help a fellow alcoholic. He said it was part of step 12. I wanted to butt in and say the only problem is I'm not an alcoholic but the guy is so genuine. Also, I didn't do that because we previously have bonded while he drove me back from the early bird blasting EDM music. He's a major DJ so that's a plus. I accepted his kind offer and agreed to call him every day. I promptly called the next day to no answer and a full voice box. Swell start to the whole "sober" friendship.

Today is a Wednesday, so it's spirituality day at the hill. At open mica or creative spirituality or hippy time in layman terms, I made a game time decision to share my poem "Sativa" about the brotherhood we've created. I wasn't nervous or scared, I read my words eloquently and then left the podium with appraise and approval and eventually fist bumps from the boys. By the way, check out the epilogue or just flip to the last page of the book to read the poem. Go do it now actually while its fresh in your head, you know, its better like that.

I than moseyed my way down to meditation where I was excited to get my dose of serenity and relaxation. I was on the tired side so I looked forward to that post meditation refreshingly awake feeling. The problem was I underestimated how tired I was. My deep breathing became deep sleep breathing and before I knew it, I was in REM sleep. Next thing I remember is drool hanging from my mouth and being shaken awake. I slept so long even the instructor was gone. I got that well rested feeling but not the conventional meditative way, guess the end justifies the means.

The only other noteworthy moment of my day came from a personal share I made at the nightly AA meeting. The speaker spoke about themes of despair, suicide and unmanageability. I decided to share something I've never told anyone. Brace yourself, this gets dark. I spoke about my depressive episode during my first semester in Madison. During pledging, I never contemplated killing myself because you know, that looks bad on me, but I had thoughts, dark thoughts. I shared that I stopped looking when I crossed the street. I wanted a bus to just take me out some days or someone to stab or shoot me in the late hours of the nights. Thank god that moment never came to pass and that bus never arrived. Also I am thankful there are no cars allowed on State Street.

DAY 16

My day again started with optimism and positivity. Everyday my mind encounters a daily reprieve of madness and insanity. I again sat next to my DJ homie and he helped and always does ease my growing but curbing anxiety. He sold me a pack of cigarettes so I didn't need to annoy the driver to stop at a gas station. At this point I was doing ok but this past and things turned dark and potentially fatal.

I was told that my social worker had my journal so I went over to retrieve it, all benign behavior, but I ran into my OG doctor and things took a vertical nosedive. I had many questions for him, even though I lied and told him I had only one so he would see me. I asked about the side effects of my drugs and his answers included weight gain and hair loss. Fantastic. Now onto my left calf, ever since an altercation between five bouncers at a strip club, it has caused me tremendous pain and discomfort. My doc told me I needed an ultrasound because the results were indeed quite important to my health. He gave me two options: I have a hematoma or a blood clot. The latter, he said, could be fatal if that clot transported to organs such as my lungs or heart. Well happy fucking New Year's Eve! Golden Hill has taught me the skill to prepare for the worst and that broke me down near tears. Fatal?!? Well that's the first time I've heard that word directed to me from a certified doctor. I was now damn near a panic attack.

I tried my very best to remain calm and block that fatal option. Teflon mind right? I immediately came back to the house to talk to my house leader. He did his very best to calm me down but just like a manic episode, at this point his efforts were futile, nothing could stop this. My breathing turned to hyperventilating. 0 to 100 real quick. I turned to my higher power and for the first time turned to my version of God.

Dear higher power, please look after me in a time of need, give me strength to face this in sobriety and wisdom to rationalize my diagnosis. Please, I want to live, I deserve it, I don't want to die. I haven't come close to accomplishing my life goal. Please, please, please let karma look after me today, take into factor my strength and recent courageous behavior. I want to help others and I can't do that if I'm dead. Stay strong, we can do this together. I'm currently 26 days sober. I will make a promise to you to make it to day 60 if you allow it. Let me live fast and die last. I don't think that's too much to ask of you, I've never asked for anything. I NEED you now. Please guide me. I seek it, want it and need it tremendously today. Let me live.

After talking to my Dad, the doc, he did his best to curb my anxiety. I'm going to the hospital today and will see what God has in store for me. My higher power has reached out to me through music. This isn't the first time I've felt like this. It's like he/she or force of nature is speaking to me through the songs he puts on through my shuffled playlist. In my panic, he eased my soul by playing "bright side of life" by Rebelution and "Karma" by Clear Conscience and "Everyday Struggle" by Biggie. The lyrics are too similar to my conscious to be coincidence. Higher power, thank you for the appropriate songs to ease my madness.

I get to the hospital and they ask me some preliminary questions: "Are you a student?" "Yes, I'm in a rehab School". "Do you have Ebola?" "No, but I tend to catch mania pretty easily". I don't think she was nearly as amused as I was. When I finally got in to see the very pretty ultrasound nurse, I was anxious to see the results. The process was actually quite intriguing. I got to hear the sound of my blood being pumped throughout my leg; it was actually quite spiritual in a sense. Finally, the consensus: I'm bipolar. Wait, wrong doctor. The actual consensus was no blood clot, just a mass of internal bleeding. Just more internal issues, I was happy to hear this one didn't have to do with my internal inclination and predisposition to mania. I could deal with that. Guess it wasn't my time to go. Oh yeah, fuck, I foxhole prayed to my higher power that if I lived I would make it sober to 60 days. Well guess I'll be doing that now. All for the better, and plus, I'll get that shiny AA chip for making it that long.

We just had alumni night at the Hill and the speaker was joyous and personable. I shared about my day and how it was the epitome of bipolar fluctuations in mood, even though I'm stable. I felt the complete array of emotions: I laughed, I cried, I prayed, I was arrogant. At the end of the day I'm stable and that's normal. Ups and downs will occur naturally, it's just important to remain conscious of your emotions and regulate them back to normal stability. After my share, I felt the natural release of tension; I could tell the speaker was proud of me fighting the stigma that men don't show emotion. Damn right I show emotion, I'm an emotional guy, I'm bipolar, it all makes sense.

My day was tremendously enhanced by my parent's presence. Today was a perfect example of their unshaken support. My mom took me to the hospital and even though I was mostly engaged with my phone, she was the cute bubbly endearingly loving Mom I knew so well as an adolescent. What I realized today is that Mom never left. Now, a word about my father. What is there even to say except everything. We had an amazing visit. We shared things we've never disclosed to each other before. I told him about my gambling and how I became a drug king pin overnight. I was honest with him and he was honest back. We reminisced about old memories together and he told me nostalgic stories of his childhood. He told me this is the healthiest he's ever seen me in so long, words can't describe how much that meant to me. We were just being real, no bullshit, it was the first time I've felt this connection in so long.

Now it's time to usher in the New Year, the year of redemption. I feel it in my mind and 100% in my heart. I reached out to some of my friends, some girls. You know you really get to see who really cares about you if they answer on NYE. Take a guess if the ex answered or not. The girl, who did answer, though, has solidified a place in my heart. I don't know which part of my heart or how much but I know she's in it. She makes me happy. We talked for 30 minutes. She told me that I make her feel like smiling. The way she eloquently stated it over the phone made my heart flutter. She said at midnight she is going to be thinking of me. Well that's about the cutest thing I've ever heard and as the ball dropped I found the feeling to be mutual. With 2016 now upon us, the whole notion of resolutions has come to fruition. The list is longer than the eldest Buddhist scrolls but I'll give a short synopsis. I am going to remain stable and ride this wave of sobriety. I am going to be calm, cool and collect and carry no resentments or hatred because that is more toxic than any drug. While we're at it, why not add to the list and state that I'm going to truly move on, for now, from my ex. To close off the year, I want to officially resign from my fratting days and hang up the gloves. While my retirement came earlier than expected, I couldn't be happier with the decision. It's time to start the next chapter with a blank piece of paper and a stable head on my shoulders. 2016 is the year of Teddy Twoface, hope the world is prepared and fuck em' if they're not.

DAY 17

Happy New Year to Teddy, and since you're talking in the third person, If I had any doubts left if I'm just a tad bit insane, it's solidified now. Way to start the New Year on a brilliant note. To just continue with the unintellectual theme, I was taking my first shit of the New Year and I just had this overwhelming rush of serenity. I did not rush it, just for those minutes I appreciated everything around me: the sink, the shower, the toilet and most importantly myself. I've grown to love the new, reborn me. I went back to my roots. In high school, I had so many hobbies. I have started to write again with a semi-manic fever, I have a passion for photography again and I play lacrosse at Wisconsin. In the words of one of my boys, "I love thyself".

An unknown man approached me after one of my shares and stated, "I want you to write this down". I obliged. He said to me, "It's better to be twisted and untwisted than to be never twisted at all." Wow. It just caught me off guard because that quote encapsulates my entire existence. Yeah I'm twisted, Fuck yeah I am. I'd choose this life 99 out of 100 times compared to the boring, white rice life. That one percent represents the guilt I still have from all the people I hurt during my manic episodes.

I got to make one very important amend today on my day pass from Golden Hill. At 12:51, she walked into the same deli we used to get sandwiches together after school. This girl is my ex. We hugged and I felt instant gratification because I knew I would finally get my chance to make things right. We chatted over coffee and as time passed, I could see her slowly warming up to me. That connection was still there, although it had been dead for so long. After giving it mouth to mouth, it's an analogy, relax, I started to make her laugh, as some things never change. I gave her a mango chap stick as we shared between us a collection of chap sticks. I know that when she uses it I'll be in her mind, a benign and yet undeniable symbol of what we once shared.

Next, I headed home. Ah, the ol' crib. First order of business is to strip down the exterior of my bedroom because it was time for a clean slate. I redecorated with artwork I made in the psych ward. In hindsight that was probably not the best idea but it looks fucking cool. Then I went to the basement, the old trap house. There she was my bong, that big fucker. I just stared back at it. It looked straight back. I touched it, moved it into storage and that was that. I'm too strong for that petty mind game. I didn't want to use it, didn't want to get high; it just didn't trigger anything even though it should have. Shortly after, one of my best friends came to visit. It was amazing to see him after so long and I could feel that the feeling was mutual. We played darts, Halo 5 and listened to Mac Miller. If heaven could be on Earth, which I do believe it can be, I was at the epicenter. I could be sober and be this happy, no bullshit. It was a needed revelation. Another revelation I had that day was I don't really like texting; it truly does take you out of the present moment. This year I'll be way more conscious of my phone usage.

My day culminated in a beautiful family sushi dinner. I was so grateful for the food and even more for my family's positive presence. My brother gave me two beaded bracelets, one signifying manic-depressive illness and another all-black one that signifies truth. Way to go bro, we're taking the first steps to rebuilding our once unbreakable bond.

Before I knew it, it was time to go back to Sativa House and I found myself physically, mentally and spiritually prepared. I even was excited, excited to see the boys. I missed the contagious laughter and the reprieve of externally driven anxiety. Wow, I really am insane, I was excited to go back to rehab and I'm damn proud of that fact.

DAY 18

M y day started off magically, in more ways than one. It started with legitimate "magic". One of my wiser and older Sativa friends showed me a couple of card tricks he has mastered over the years. He even broke the golden rule of magic and showed me sleight of hand and the mathematics behind the tricks. Don't worry, I still believe in the power of magic I just now know how those sly dogs pull it off. Shortly after, I went outside to face the pleasure of the present shining sun. I sat down alone and sparked one and listened to the ambience of the early brisk morning. Some of my boys came out after a short while to join my jovial bliss. What a start to a beautiful day.

In one of our workshops today we fixated on co-dependence. It was highly enjoyable and even more enlightening, so many nuggets of wisdom my pen couldn't keep up. The brilliant staff member who ran it had so much knowledge to impart on us. She started off with discussing emotions and how important it was to be aware of them and why and who effects them. She astutely pointed out that the people in our close circle have the greatest capability of fucking with our emotional spectrum. This was an important fact to know because it has been the ones closest to me that have had the most emotional impact on me, for better or for worse.

We then segued into discussing the stigma behind mental illness. For people who don't have it's impossible for them to understand let alone show genuine empathy. It's like trying to describe the color blue to a blind person. It's just fucking blue. It's like trying to explain the pain of being shot to a white kid in Westchester; they're more than likely not going to understand.

We then delved into the main discussion of co-dependency. I was already interested because I'm highly aware that I used to be extremely dependent on my high school girlfriend. We both were. We would often isolate ourselves and live in a happy fictional fantasy world. The result was ultimately a disability in self-identification. We were inseparable, it was like having a sandwich with just peanut butter or just jelly, and you just didn't have one without the other. I am so grateful to be able to see this now because it has allowed me to discover aspects of who I really am.

Speaking of old relationships and friends, one of my long lost girl friends came to visit me today. It was great to rekindle. It's funny because she admitted that in high school she never thought we would be friends. See what doors you close when you isolate yourself. I actually have no regrets; I loved closing my bedroom door with my ex. Did I mention she was a model back then? Off topic but needed to be said. It was beautiful to walk the grounds with my friend and just talk. We both have complicated histories, lots of demons in our closets so it was refreshing taking turns cleaning out painful old memories. It was mutually healthy and entertaining in a twisted way. Her visit crystallized the importance of letting go and letting time heal emotional wounds because you never know whom you can become close with when you have an open mind and an open heart.

Lastly, to close out my very interesting day, I opened my metaphorically closed door. It started with the in house speaker. We discussed the 12 steps and I had a momentary lapse in judgment. It stemmed from confusion. I'm going to disclose the entirety of my journal entry notes so you can really see the full mentality switch I endured in the span of just two hours. I wrote:

> I have a problem with the 12 steps because I'm here for a different reason than everyone else, I'm bipolar. I am not powerless to alcohol or even weed so I can't get past step one. Step two I can fuck with. When you take out God and replace my higher power with nature, the sun, the moon, and the stars, it makes sense but step three can go fuck itself. It's total bullshit. I won't "turn my will and life over to the care of God", not to this holy God or anyone for that fact. It's my strength and courage that has gotten me to this point. Why would I turn it over, my hard work, to a faceless man in the sky?"

Whoa there cowboy, as you can see, I went on this emotional rant. It can't be a coincidence that the next AA meeting, run by my now pissed off sponsor because I yet again forgot to call him, is about the fucking 12 steps. I shared with him and the group the exact rant I previously emphatically gave. He just stared back at me. I could feel him disagreeing with my every word but he remained silent. It took 15 minutes for me to raise my hand again and say I had some revisions to make from my previous statements. I expressed to him and the entire room that I abused drugs as a kid, when I was depressed, when I was stable, and most definitely when I was clinically insane. I ended my share with explicitly stating, "I AM AN ADDICT", and then my sponsor smiled. I was so dumb at 18; I'm 19 now and it's time to face the absolute truth. I proclaim truth is the only language I speak so here it goes.

Hi, my name is Teddy Twoface and I am a bipolar addict. That's the truth. Call a spade a spade motherfuckers.

DAY 19

Why is it that the start of every good beautiful day can't be maintained for the duration of the day? It is becoming apparent that nothing I do is good enough for this world. My parents arrive and we immediately start fighting about my aftercare. I offer to live at home, at a sober house, get a job, get two jobs, take classes, take online classes and none of it seems good enough. I want to implode. We then go to the library to look into Wisconsin online courses and I receive an email saying I've been kicked out of the university for a low GPA. I got a fucking D in a 1 credit music course because I missed the final because my parents pulled me from school the week before finals, even though I warned them of the detrimental academic effects it would cause but that clearly didn't mean shit. Sorry Wisconsin, I was unable to be a student because my frat was making me vomit every other day for a semester and then I experienced my first dose of mania during the second. Do I fucking deserve this? I'll answer this question and this one I'll answer correctly, no. I've suffered enough. It is time I see some fucking positives in this life. Life is beautiful? La vita e' bella?

Nah, all I see is pain and unfair treatment of the mentally ill. I am smarter than half the students at this school; sorry my GPA can't reflect that. Life's a bitch; Nas knew exactly what he was talking about.

Every time I'm sucker punched with bad news, I'm smacked with a message, this time it had a silver lining, literally. Directly after hearing from Wisconsin our next group was cinema therapy where we watched "Silver Lining's Playbook." If you haven't seen it, first off, go fucking see it because it's fantastic. If you haven't, I'll give my readers a little insight on this masterpiece. It's about Bradley Cooper's character battling his bipolar and learning to cope with it and eventually learn to love again. He's able to do so by having an open mind and clearly open eyes because he meets and gets to know Jennifer Lawrence's amazing character. He uses the mantra "excelsior" in times of manic panic. This movie is my life in a movie and watching it gives me shivers down my spine in both good and scary ways. My spirit animal is Bradley Cooper's character; actually it's a blend of him, Jax Teller and Tyler Durden. Life is all about finding positivity in negativity and always searching for that silver lining no matter how many times life sucker punches you in the gut.

DAY 20

Everyday I recover from insanity I become stronger. The future, the palpable sensation of stability, becomes a realistic lifestyle, not a dream I escape to when I close my eyes at the end of a long day.

Since we're discussing energy, aka the force, I'm going to George Lucas this day and start at the end and work forward. I ended today looking up at the vast night sky. I didn't care that it was only 9 degrees; I needed to see my higher power, G.O.D, the great outdoors. After such an empowering NA meeting, I had this newfound appreciation for this world and myself. Only a powerful speaker can have a powerful profound effect on oneself. This speaker tonight spoke from the heart that's why I believe I felt it in my heart. It wasn't his story that empowered me, although it did, it was the message he was conveying to us all. It was like he was individually going around and giving us each a warm hug; his words made me feel loved and appreciated. It was such an endearing trait. This was the one meeting in all my 20 days that I didn't want to end. This man had so much wisdom I wanted to soak it all in like a sponge but alas, even after I spoke with him alone after the meeting and physically got that hug, I was pulled back to Scativa for our evening wrap up. This guys "thing" is actually giving individual hugs. Who fucking knew! My attitude was gratitude and I owe that to this man.

Earlier in the day in one of my groups, we did a powerful exercise called psychodrama. It works by envisioning two paths in the form of chairs: one symbolizing 6 months then two years in the wrong direction vice versa in the right direction. The right direction is defined by following "the program". I volunteered first because I knew I would gain much from this. At each checkpoint, you are asked to describe how your life is going. My dark path, when described aloud, sounded miserable. It included not taking my medication, not being allowed to go back to Wisconsin, doing drugs, having a broken family dynamic, lying, cheating, and the accumulation of slipping back into mania and returning to my favorite psych ward. Fuck that shit. My other path sounded exponentially more fun and fulfilling. It included stability, trust, Wisconsin, a successful business, a successful writing career, healthy sexual relationships and giving back to my fellow psychotics and most importantly loving myself. After acting out both scenarios, it was abundantly clear which path I desperately wanted. I want the suffering to end and I want the joy to return and stay for a lifetime. I would give it all up, anything that got in the way, in order to achieve this way of life. The beautiful thing is I have the tools and knowledge to obtain it.

Which brings me back to the beginning. Today was my 30th day of sobriety. In AA and in life that's a momentous milestone. As I walked up to collect my 30-day coin I was overcome with emotion. You are told to say a few words after and that I did. I told the early bird crowd, packed with fellow addicts, that I didn't think this day would be achievable. In high school I couldn't imagine going one week clean and in college I couldn't fathom going just 24 hours.

It was due to the relentless support of my peers, now brothers and sisters in sobriety that I was able to achieve this milestone. The applause, for a moment, was near deafening and it left my heart throbbing of pride for hours to come. This is just a slight peer into the window of the overwhelming support I receive on a daily basis.

With 30 days of sobriety under my belt, it has become clear that we must inhale both pain and beauty life provides us. It is then we are able to see both perspectives, to be able to see and find that silver lining in the sometimes-overwhelming negativity this life provides us. Life is a journey where the destination is irrelevant. It is the nuggets of wisdom we pick up along the way that makes this harsh world tolerable. Life is knowing that this world is greater than you. I am a compilation of my loved ones; I am not a single entity. If I choose the dark path and decide to descend into the depths of hell, I'll have my friends and family attached to the chariot but this will not be the case. I am choosing the path of the program and in doing so I'll be chasing happiness, my ultimate goal.

DAY 21

"One can have no smaller or greater mastery than mastery of oneself"

– Leonardo Da Vinci.

"Can you let me fucking talk now"

– Teddy Twoface

Ah, the great juxtaposition of quotes encapsulates my day and really my entire journey here. I had my family meeting today with my parents, doctor and social worker and it was a bipolar glass box of emotions. Before things turned south, both my parents acknowledged how far I've come including my willingness to take medication and my utmost participation in the program as a whole. However, with discharge creeping up, so many pieces of the puzzle have yet to be put in place. That was the root of some of the arguing. The main contributing factors were the disapproval of re-vamping my unborn company and my unpublished book. I chose to describe these dreams of mine in such a manner to convey to you that I still very much knew they were works in progress but how do you ever get something accomplished if you don't steadily put in daily effort? I know they are grandiose ideas; the problem is so do my parents. Convinced they were born out of mania, they see these demon spawn ideas as destined to destroy me. It's quite the contrary parents: they are going to be the key to my future. Perhaps that's why my mom over the phone, later in the day, said to me that regardless of what the professionals say, if this is what is going to make me happy, she supported my efforts. She even told me to write it in my journal, quite emphatically I might add. I almost couldn't believe my ears. Wait what did she say? She supports my dreams and aspirations? But like, in the room two hours ago before you were saying…fuck it, it doesn't matter it was said and now it shall be true. This really shouldn't have been a surprise to me. This is my damn mother were talking about: the strongest, the wisest and most insightful human I've ever known. Damn, was I proud to be her son.

After that, my spirits were lifted and I was impromptu visited by my boy Chris, the same Chris who is the DJ. I was so grateful and honored that he took time out of his day to come chill and talk to me. He had no obligation to do so, he can't sponsor anyone because he doesn't have enough sobriety days under his belt but that's all politics. The connection we have goes beyond sponsor-ship. He is my friend, my brother and family. Someone I could relate to and confide in and plus I found out he was 19! No fucking wonder we connected and had so much in common. What we are doing for each other is beautiful. Through friendship and laughter we are both keeping each other clean. Even though were the same age, I value his word like it was coming from the mouth of a long time AA vet. He told me the importance of self-searching because when you are sober you find you have a lot less true friends than you originally thought. He spoke so wisely. We were both two 19 year olds, aged by the rough journey of life. We were greater than our expected comprehension. We are the ones that have so much left to learn but we know one subject quite well: ourselves. "One can have no smaller or greater mastery than mastery of oneself". This is the truth. Mr. Da Vinci, Chris and I hear you loud and clear.

ENLIGHTENMENT: WEEK 4

DAY 22

You know when a baby learns to walk and he tries and to make his first steps and fails? You know it, you expect it, and you allow it. Then the baby gets up and tries again and the same result but eventually he gets a couple steps in then collapses, maybe even harder than the first time he tried. This has been my life up until this point except I'm the bipolar addict baby. I've had one really bad manic episode, drug-induced they thought, and I fell. Then I tried again in the same environment, that endearing drowning booze state of Wisconsin, and I fell again but this time it was much harder. Not because of the mental manic state I reached, but because I had the tools to prevent it. I did the same things expecting a different outcome. That's insanity on top of pre-existing insanity. This long convoluted metaphor has a purpose. My falling down repetitively has led me here. I have the choice to dust myself off and try again and I'm here to tell you I've successfully taken my first baby steps in my long life of tough situations regarding sobriety.

It's my best college friend Jake's, birthday, and his party is around the time I get out of rehab. I wanted so desperately to see him, to see all my Wisco ladies and gents, to celebrate and really test myself. Even my parents were entertaining the idea. I brought it up in an in house AA meeting with a particular hard-nosed, tough love speaker. I knew the answer he was going to give before I even phrased my dilemma. The answer was obviously don't go to the fucking party. He also pointed out that a true friend wouldn't put me in that situation fresh out of rehab. He looked me dead in the eyes and said, "We're going to come to a conclusion right now, are you going to go to the party?" The answer just poured out of me, "No". I have so much respect for this man for what he pointed out in me. I can do this. Now I can't credit this conclusion all to this man because prior to the meeting I called Jake about coming and he flat out said he didn't think it was a good idea but I didn't yet understand why. Immediately after the meeting I called him and told him I shouldn't go and he said how truly proud he was of me for making that choice. Jake is seriously one of the best kids I know. You know him. The funny kid who always puts everyone's problems before his own. He said he would round up the pledge class and drive down to me for dinner just to see me. I was in tears; I am in tears now as I write this because the amount of love I have for this little guy is unconditional. He would jump off a cliff first to scope it out to make sure it was safe for me. Ya just can't find kids like him anymore.

Not to be an AA slogan slut but step 6 was the topic of the early bird this morning. It talks about ridding ourselves of our impurities, our defects. This can be frightening to highlight your faults at first because you think if you strip away your faults, your drugging, your "cool side", you will be left with nothing. That is false. False friends come from failure to personally purify yourself. Nobody can to this for you, as it is an individual effort. A facade of character attracts the wrong crowd. So lets say you believe that if you take away all your character defects you'll be left empty. In reality you are not empty but quite the opposite, you are left with the gems of your personality, the true character traits, the ones you had all that time before "life got life-y" and addiction plagued you. True friends love you for the gems. Jake is my best friend and he loves me because of my gems not the pretense of a deceased frat star.

DAY 23

You're not responsible for your first thought of the day but Hank sure as fuck held me accountable and I'm glad he did. I didn't want to go to the early bird because, I don't know, I was tired? Tired physically? Tired of the constant AA meetings? Whatever the case may be Hank wasn't buying it. He gave me a small dose of tough love saying it shows a sign of weakness. He was right. So, sleepy eyed I went and got dressed, still hung over from my night meds, bumping into closet doors but I eventually stumbled my way over to the coffee pot for the one stimulant my body is allowed to consume. I'm so grateful I went because in the middle of a big book reading, a particularly boring one, the same in house speaker that I had the intellectual spar about going to the party came over to me and whispered, "Did you make the call?" I said, "Yes sir." He firmly shook my hand and patted me on the back. The sensation of his lingering handshake left my hand tingling for minutes. I never felt that before, it was the tingles of residual pride. Oh and by the way I got dumped today. It was the first time I've ever been dumped. My fucking sponsor left my ass and it was after I called him telling him how good my day was going! I quickly hung up the phone because I couldn't contain my laughter. Best break up in history.

Two amazing people visited today and consoled my broken heart. Andrew and Reid. Both on the shorter side, Andrew has that cool haircut where it's shaved on the sides and long on the top. With his growing maturity, his look has become one of cool European. Reid, with his contagious laugh, is the little brother I never had. A year younger than me, I've tried to impart some wisdom and I pray he's learned from my faults. He has this cool snowboarder look to him. With a strong attitude, I know he's ready for pledging. He's going to take no shits and give no fucks. He'll be loved and adored and in response people will follow his lead. He is a leader or at least has the potential to become one. Our NA speaker, amazing voice, powerful and strong, talked about how you couldn't go back to your drug buddies. I wanted, just for a second, to get up and rock the old dude. He's up there preaching while he has no idea about my two day one pals. Yeah, we used to smoke together, like a lot, like everyday, but do you expect me to cut them out just because of that? I won't slap a label on them and perceive them as a negative influence. I played flag football when I was 12 with Andrew and have been on countless lacrosse teams with Reid. They were behind me in the early days, behind me when I was a middle school skateboard punk, behind me when I was a trippy stoner in high school, behind me when I was a druggy college freshman, behind me when I lost my mind, behind me when I couldn't get out of my bed crippled with depression and they sure as fuck are behind me in sobriety if that's the path I choose because since day one they want their best friend to be happy and healthy. That's a beautiful thing man, a beautiful thing. Andy, Reid, you have my unwavering unconditional love. Never forget that.

DAY 24

D enial: a reoccurring theme through out anyone's journey in
life. In mine, it's been a prevalent one. Diagnosed with two
cunning diseases you can almost add denial as a third but this one
is curable. Through AA and NA and the following fellowship, I've
eradicated denial from my life. I just recently acknowledged my
consistent denial that I was over my high school sweetheart. I am
proud to say I've crossed out her number on my sheet of contacts.
I did this for both our sanities. I know, in my heart, even though
she repetitively hasn't shown her support through words or phone
calls, she will always support me. I wanted to call her and ask her
about a specific suspect new man in her life but I realized it was
irrelevant. We are friends now and that's all that truly matters. If
she's happy, I'm happy and more than likely than not I'm way more
happy.

To segue perfectly into the next portion of my day I asked an
in house speaker about dating after discharge. He said to not get
into a heavy, heart consuming relationship because it could spark
a relapse. He even went as far to tell me to use my looks and be

a stud with "fuck buddies". Fuck buddies! This advice I couldn't refute. Hey, they tell you to follow the program so I guess I would be doing myself a disservice if I didn't listen to the professionals.

Denial of my diseases won't accomplish anything and I have big things to accomplish. I am not in denial anymore. Not in any aspect of my life and I truly have never been happier. I am a crazy, bipolar kid predisposed to get addicted to not one but all things. It's my personality. Henry David Thoreau once said, "In the wildness is the preservation of the world". My wildness will be used as a harmless weapon to help me achieve good, not to inflict pain on anyone and most importantly myself. I've never been so proud to be who I am. I still have much to learn about the ruthless diseases I've been dealt but I can't hope for a better past, just the capability to change my future.

DAY 25

3 5 days sober. I'm choosing to start this entry in this manner because "35" has a major familial sentimental value. My mom wore that number throughout her athletic career and my brother followed suit by wearing it throughout his lacrosse career. Then, when it was my turn, my brother literally gave me the number in the form of his old lax jersey. I was so honored. I put blood, sweat and tears in that jersey and eventually added the title captain to the jersey legacy. This day symbolizes hard work, family, determination and courage. Today I faced my day with all these attributes at my disposal.

Since I was determined this day was to be filled with positivity I started it off in such a manner. I gave my lucky cig and last menthol to my boy and real good friend for the past three and half weeks. I believe that if you want luck, you need to give luck. I'm starting to truly believe in that because literally an hour later I called a girl I'm friends with and she made an impromptu stop on her way from Maine to New York to visit me. Now that's some higher power luck coincidence baller shit if you ask me. Our visit was really just amazing; I expected it to be as we have a very unique friendship. This relationship was born in a cuckoo's nest and nurtured in a rehab facility. Now that has to be the first time in human history a friendship has started in such a manner and it's beautiful. A little back-story on her: She's bipolar like me but on the depressive side. We met in a psych ward and she has supported my recovery. That means more to me than anything. I don't care if you're a barstool smoke show or fat Amy, if you were there for me during my lowest times I'm going to have a special place in my heart for you. Since she has the tendency to be depressed and I have the tendency to go manic, we balance each other out. She is the yin to my yang. When I was with her I felt this overwhelming sensation of calm come over me. She was like living meditation. I'm not sure if that trait is likely to be found in a guy or girl. She is just another powerful example that you can always learn something about yourself through the experiences you share with another.

What I've learned through various relationships and friendships with women is the power of love and the equally strong power of hate. I want neither in my life at the moment. Such intense feelings can only distract oneself from goals such as sobriety, happiness and writing. They do make for some awfully good material to write about however. Here's how I see it: love and hate are not actually opposites, though widely believed to be. Believed by most as absolute truth, the two emotions seem to sequentially follow each other. That may be true but that doesn't make them opposites. Love and hate are intertwined and related like distant cousins. In reality, their relationship is only founded on the fact that they both require energy. There is energy to love and toxic energy to hate. Love and hate, similar, yet so different, can be lumped together. The true opposite lies in indifference. Indifference requires no energy. It is just a state of the absence of emotion. Both love and hate are emotionally charged feelings. Both, however, have the capability to ruin and suck the joy out of ones life. This is the root of my wary caution to engage in either at the present moment. It's a healthy fear but not a permanent one.

Now that my philosophical debate between said emotions is done we can discuss the enlightenment I reached at tonight's AA meeting. My ex-sponsor was running it so I intuitively knew it was both going to be motivational, educational and part giving me shit out of love. Through his story and wisdom he got me to really admit aloud that I could at least potentially be an alcoholic. I am an addict. That much has been established. Alcohol is a drug. Drugs are drugs. Addicts get addicted to drugs. You see the reasoning I'm going for here? Labels don't mean shit. What really matters is the recovery aspect of the journey. The addiction and suffering is the heinous part, the beauty lies in the recovery. Suffering is to live. To live is to suffer but to live is to find meaning in the suffering. Not only will I survive, but also I will thrive and that is the most beautiful thing of all.

DAY 26

I'm at a loss of words. Actually no I'm fucking not, I have plenty to say. I have been feverishly reading "An Unquiet Mind" by Kay Jamison and the parallels are frightening in an intellectual enlighteningly way. I was once on high doses, toxic levels, of lithium and I felt every side effect Jamison writes about. I want to publically denounce my old psychiatrist and state the following: I fucking hate you. You almost put me in such a depressive state that I wanted to kill myself. What an uneducated scumbag. Did he not read Kay's book?!? I was describing, word for word, the negative side effects and it didn't matter. He perceived me as insane and was adamant about not lowering my dose. My blood pressure is spiking with the painful thoughts of this very low time in my life.

With high blood pressure and a sense of rage, I called the one girl I knew could talk me out of rage, Tami. She is a girl I met in Wisconsin. We have this relationship like no other. Both traumatized by previous "love" affairs or really just me since she refuses to think so. Regardless, we are able to connect on a much deeper, harder level. Sometimes I can understand her deep emotions by just the way she looks at me. That stare, is indescribable and it does hit me in the heart, for better or worse. She has been there every step of the way. She calmed me down during our formal when I was hypo manic and pissed we missed the cruise. She was the only person to this day that has been able to calm me when I was in this heightened state. She now supports my recovery mentally, spiritually and most definitely physically. I truly can't thank this girl enough. We have these deep philosophical talks on the phone basically every night. She makes me laugh and feel the whole spectrum of emotions, again for better or for worse. I've never met a girl like her, red haired, empowered, wise, creative as fuck and knows more about football and cars than me. That would piss some guys off; I think it's unique. She is the one that is not quite like the others and that is what attracts me to her the most.

Later in the day, we had one of the most comical in house AA meetings in Scativa history. This old dude starts off by saying he has the flu and proceeds to shake everyone's hands. Classic. After the meeting we all frantically pass around the hand sanitizer but this wasn't what got everyone in tears. His agenda was to go around the room and ask for everyone's story on how they got there. It was evident by the second person that this guy just wasn't all there. When he got to me, I started to delve into my story. How I was introduced to drugs at a young age and how good my high school life was and how my life got flipped upside down when I entered college. I really got into the details of it all, I'm not quite sure why I was so in depth but I was. When I talked about my depressive and manic episodes he interrupted and told me I probably don't have bipolar. Hmm. I was stunned. I went deeper into my manic stories but right in the middle he goes, "You definitely don't have bipolar". The room lost it. Two of my boys had to excuse themselves because they were laughing too hard. They weren't laughing at me; actually they kind of were because I'm now trying to convince this old fuck I'm bipolar. Most of the laughter was due to the obvious arrogance of this guy. In some ways it was the funniest thing of all time and everyone was streaming tears. Yo, old fuck, as much as it would be super chill to not have this life threatening illness, I have it and am quite aware of it. I'm not going to ignore the diagnosis of ten or more doctors but thanks for the fleeting false hope old flu festering fuck. Lucky I'm a calm dude now or I would have verbally destroyed this guy. That is the beauty of writing a book; I can do it all right here. So again, fuck you, you unqualified, unintelligent, decaying old shit. All those drugs clearly had a major impact on your ability to perceive the even most obvious of things: I'm insane!

If it isn't clear by this entry I have some trust issues with doctors, psychiatrists, therapists and now I can add old dudes in AA to the list.

DAY 27

Last night I did something I've never done before. I looked up at the night sky and prayed. I don't know whom I was praying to or if anyone was listening but I did it. Looking up at the shining stars, wishing I could be up in the high atmosphere, flying amongst the plants in a peaceful coexistence. I said a few words along the lines of, "Dear higher power, thank you for giving me this second shot at life, for the very existence of the this enlightening, mystical establishment". The Hill has blown away my expectations and shattered my previous conceptions of mental and spiritual power. I truly feel like an enlightened individual. Up until today, everyday when we would close out meetings with the serenity prayer, I would leave the first word out: god. I don't do that anymore. It's all relative and now having a firm ideology and foundation in spirituality, I am comfortable including the word in the prayer. Regardless of my personal beliefs in the existence of a religious God, I am now able to bypass that once spiritual blockade and see the bigger picture. It is our higher power that can help restore us to sanity and I can use all the help I can get in that department.

So today was the first part of the family program. It's where the parents spend two days prior learning about what the patients have learned and then the next two days are emotionally charged where the parents and patients come together to confront and talk about underlying issues of the past and present. Most of the patients dread these days for all sorts of reasons. Anxiety spikes and PRNs (as needed medications) are popped like candy. For me, I was not nervous. The perks of being honest are that when you are put in situations like this, the pain of coming clean is already completed. Mom and I murked it. We were this dynamic duo, both trying to bring levity to the stressful environment. I guess the deranged apple doesn't fall far from the stable tree. People were coming up to me saying how "mushy" my mom and I looked. I seized every opportunity to show genuine affection because I still harbor guilt from the acidic words I once said in my manic stages of my life. At the end we went around the circle and shared what we learned. When it got to me I already had tears in my eyes. I thanked my Mom for her unconditional love and support and how moving forward days would be filled with light rather than darkness. With tears streaming down my face, I kissed her head and felt the connection only a mother and son can have. When I later called my Dad who couldn't make it due to work he said my mom was gushing over the way I handled myself and that her feet were not on the floor due to pure elation. That left a smile on my face for the duration of the day.

DAY 28

Ah the last day. Hoorah, feeling like Marky Mark in Lone Survivor right now. I came in fighting and now leaving, lone wolf, back to fight the war of reality. I'm not scared, anxious or nervous. I am a hard bodied, hairy-chested, rootin, shootin, parachutin bipolar addict. I'm fit for battle. Bring it on. There is no sky to high or sea too rough. I anticipate and encourage one hell of a good gunfight. Hit me with all the triggers you got. If you are feeling like jumping, jump, because this survivor has been there, done that and is coming back for all you got. Life won't derail me from my ultimate goal, serenity and peace. I'd like to see that motherfucker try.

The second part of the family program started off rocky. I was exhausted from staying up late watching the college national final game, which was a dope game I must say, and I got to spend it with Jake on his last night. I have so much love for that Jesse Pinkman sounding motherfucker. I went to the early bird as well so by the time it was 10 in the morning I was spent and to top it off they fucked up my meds so I couldn't get my klonopin. On the one damn day I truly needed it are you kidding! I felt irritation, so before my agitation became a risk to all around me, I got a tap on my back with a message saying my meds were ready. Holla-fucking-lujah. The fresh air, dose of calmness and use of DBT skills allowed me to return to the meeting ready for action. I kissed my mom and we got back to work. Since we've been through hell and back already, we were able to sit back and soak in the stories of others and really try to help some people through moments of grief. I could see how amazing my mom was at her job because she was doing it in front of my eyes. She couldn't help it; the therapist in her is always there. I cried serious tears in that room. Not anything to do with my family and I but from the stories and the visible pain of some of the parents and my friends. It humbled me and made me grateful for my perfectly imperfect family.

My last AA meeting at the Hill was eerily perfect. It was an outsiders meeting meaning other people could attend. All my boys from the early bird were there, Jake came back for it, Chris the Dj and countless others were there. Most hysterical was my ex sponsor who still saved (and insisted I sit in) a front row seat next to him. I humbly accepted. Now the real comical part of the meeting was the speaker was the same lady who failed out of Wisconsin. When she said that part of the story and also added that she hated it there, she pointed me out and the whole room was in an uproar. She said, "I was a fuck up and never went to class and I assume you weren't too different because you're here". Roasted, checkmate. I said she hit the nail on the head. Her topic of discussion was honesty. I gave my last share and put my whole soul in it. I said it was my last day and I came in a compulsive liar, telling my parents everything they wanted to hear. Of course I'm going to class and obviously my grades are great! Through this program I've learned to speak rigorous truths, to be a man, a man that can be accountable for his actions. I do not believe in coincidences anymore because that meeting, this closing of my journey was meant to end like this.

I concluded my share with one line, "when I do go back to school, I'm going back with the lessons I've learned here and the support of my family."

The best part of my day has finally arrived: the roast. This is the Scativa House tradition of making jokes and sending love to your departing homie. I was honored to be elected mayor of the house for my last few days here, truly a humbling notion. My boys had me in tears, tears of genuine laughter. Lines being dropped that they didn't get a celebrity but they got to live with the bipolar Justin Timberlake and how I'm the 19 year old 90 year old with the way I talk in spiritual lingo. Also, they gave humbling advice for the future that syphilis is totally treatable and a stud like me shouldn't go out like that. By this point, my ribs hurt from laughing so hard. In response, I gave my last individual roast of everyone mixed in with some philosophical wisdom. I could feel everybody truly listening and that experience is one I'll never forget. People 10, 20, 30 years older than me telling me they've learned so much about themselves through interactions with me was extremely gratifying. Encouraged by the boys, they told me to sign the "butt hutt" (the designated smoking gazebo) as all mayors have in terms past. I decided to really leave my legacy. Right above Jake's, I signed "Manic mayor Teddy Twoface" and left the dates of my term and of course a yin and yang. I am proud of my physical mark left for future generations to see but more importantly proud of the memories we collectively created. To them I'm not some crazy manic frat star but a wise young man who worked his ass off the day I checked into admissions. That is the legacy I will leave behind, the legacy of Teddy Twoface.

EPILOGUE

Well there you have it, a small look into a chaotic journey of a growing man finding himself. One chapter ends and a new one seamlessly starts. Let it be clear that this is just small piece of my life, one snippet, one frame, on a roll of film that is my life. I have only shared the journey of my 28 days in rehab. There is still so much of the story left untold like how did I get there? How did a kid who had it all end up in a psych ward not once but twice? All your questions will be answered in the form of a prequel explaining my upbringing and my journey through high school and college. The insanity will continue and this is just the start of the sharing of stories. It is a therapeutic way for me to unleash the vast emotions contained in my brain. It also serves as a vehicle to spark conversation about mental illness and addiction. Through my stories, I am attempting to tap into the mainstream and help fight the stigma behind my disease. Please read and share my message, if you know someone with bipolar or addiction tell them to read my short book or at least tell them its going to be alright. There is a solution, a cure; to what some would say is an incurable disease. There is no need to hide in the shadows anymore. Be proud of what you have, use it as a weapon for good not evil. Bipolar energy bunnies are the ones who create the art you look at, the music you listen to and the literature you read. Be proud. Own what you have. Don't let it rule you. Harness your illness and unleash its beauty upon the world.

WORDS OF WISDOM

Quotes gathered during my 28 days in rehab

- "You're as sick as your secrets"
- "Yesterday was history tomorrow is a mystery"
- "Drugs gave me wings then took away the sky"
- "Things may not get better, but you will"
- "I'm grateful for the pain because it brought me here"
- "Dogs will bark"
- "Rome wasn't built in a day but it burnt down pretty fucking fast"
- "This too shall pass" – for Scarlett
- "Step inside a hula-hoop, that is all you have"
- "I'm locked in prison I created with the key in my pocket"
- "Older people don't get wiser, they just run out of dumb shit to do"
- "When a vending machine eats your dollar, it eats your dollar"
- "I've learned more from pain than pleasure"
- "Religion is for people afraid of hell, spirituality is for the people who've already been"
- "All that wander are not lost"
- "Smart people know what to say, wise people know when to say it"

SATIVA

Cherish the moments in Scativa
Treasure them
These friends
These brothers
Are the truth
The by products of a semi self destructive life style
Relate, identify, laugh, love
Feelings I didn't or never felt
Now feelings I feel everyday
Getting high, fake chuckles is one thing
This is not this thing
Laughter never felt so genuine
I'm technically in a fraternity
Technically have a fraternity of brothers
Technically a frat star
Nah
I am now in a brotherhood with a just cause
Banding behind sobriety
This is the truth
The only language I speak

www.ingramcontent.com/pod-product-compliance
Lightning Source LLC
Chambersburg PA
CBHW070328190526
45169CB00005B/1790